EAT YOUR FOOD AND MELT BODY FATS

Methods to eat healthly and lose weight while eating those foods you have in your kitchen.

Jenny Pearl.

Table of contents

Introduction: Unveiling The Power Of Food

In the heart of a quaint culinary haven, where aromas danced like secret lovers, a tantalizing journey unfolded. "Eat Your Food and Melt Body Fats" isn't just a book; it's a love story between you and the transformative power of food. Picture a table set with passion, where every bite whispers promises of a more vibrant you.

Meet Olivia, a culinary virtuoso, who discovered the art of crafting dishes that not only seduced taste buds but also melted away the barriers to self-love. As she stirred, sprinkled, and savored each moment in her kitchen, she realized the untold romance between food and body. This book unravels the mystery behind ingredients that caress your senses and ignite the flames of a healthier, happier you.

Join this gastronomic affair where chapters unfold like love letters. From the allure of spices to the dance of flavors in mindful eating, "Eat Your Food and Melt Body Fats" is an odyssey into the seductive world where passion on the plate becomes a catalyst for your body's enchanting transformation. Embrace the love affair; let every bite be a step towards a more enchanting you.

Chapter One

The Culinary Metamorphosis

Embark on a culinary metamorphosis with "Eat Your Food and Melt Body Fats," a gastronomic journey that transcends mere recipes. This book, a culinary chrysalis, guides you through the alchemical transformation of ingredients into agents of change.

Imagine a kitchen as your sacred laboratory, where the mundane becomes magical. The sizzle of olive oil, the fragrance of herbs – each element is a spell, woven to sculpt your body with grace. Here, food isn't just sustenance; it's the catalyst for metamorphosis.

Witness the pages unfold like a recipe-based spellbook. From enchanted smoothies that whisper promises of vitality to salads that weave a tapestry of nutrients, each chapter is a portal into a world where taste and transformation converge. The culinary metamorphosis isn't about deprivation; it's about indulging wisely, choosing ingredients that embrace you in a delicious embrace of health.

As you dive into the pages, let the culinary alchemy guide you towards a butterfly-like transformation. "Eat Your Food and Melt Body Fats" is more than a cookbook; it's the key to unlocking the enchantment within your meals, creating a symphony of flavors that orchestrates a radiant, healthier you.

Chapter Two

Flavorful Fat-Burn Recipes

Dive into a culinary symphony with "Eat Your Food and Melt Body Fats," a book that transcends ordinary recipes into a flavor-filled voyage of transformation. Imagine a kitchen as a playground of taste where each recipe is a masterpiece, meticulously crafted to elevate your health.

The first act unfolds with a zesty ballet of citrus-infused quinoa salad, where the tangy notes of lemon intertwine with the earthiness of quinoa, promising both flavor ecstasy and fat-burning prowess. Witness the savory pas de deux of garlic-roasted vegetables, a dance that elevates nutritional density while enchanting your palate.

But this gastronomic journey is more than a feast for the taste buds; it's a narrative of wellness. Indulge in the sultry tango of spicy avocado salsa atop grilled chicken, where the metabolism-boosting heat meets the creamy embrace of avocado, creating a dish that's as enticing as it is nutritious.

In the grand finale, savor the dessert duet of dark chocolate-dipped strawberries, a guilt-free indulgence that ignites the senses without compromising health. Each recipe is a chapter in the epic tale of flavor and fat-burning fusion, where your kitchen becomes the stage for a delectable revolution. "Eat Your Food and Melt Body Fats" is your passport to a world where every bite is not just a culinary delight but a step towards a healthier, more vibrant you.

Chapter Three

Taste The Transformation: Mindful Eating Practice

"Taste the Transformation: Mindful Eating Practices" in "Eat Your Food and Melt Body Fats" isn't just a chapter; it's a guide to revolutionize your relationship with food. Imagine a culinary sanctuary where every bite is a moment of mindful indulgence, unlocking the secret to a healthier you.

Picture a fork as a wand, and each bite as a spell of awareness. Dive into the first enchantment, savoring the slow, deliberate enjoyment of a succulent bite of grilled chicken, allowing each flavor note to dance on your taste buds. Feel the aliveness in each morsel, as you engage in a mindful pas de deux with a vibrant kale salad, relishing the crisp textures and earthy hues.

The chapter unfolds like a poetic narrative, inviting you to savor the poetry of a mindful bite. Indulge in the ritual of sipping a calming herbal tea between courses, a moment of serenity amidst the culinary symphony. Through mindful bites, you'll discover the transformative power of being present with your plate.

As you turn each page, "Taste the Transformation" becomes a mindful pilgrimage, reshaping not just your eating habits but your entire approach to wellness. This isn't just a culinary adventure; it's an exploration of the profound connection between mindfulness and the art of savoring life—one bite at a time.

Chapter Four

Savoring Success: Stories of Culinary Triumph.

"Savoring Success: Stories of Culinary Triumph" within "Eat Your Food and Melt Body Fats" is a narrative feast that transcends recipes, inviting you into the intimate tales of those who embraced the culinary metamorphosis. Imagine a culinary anthology where each story is a triumph, a testament to the transformative power of conscious eating.

Meet Sarah, once bound by diet culture, now relishing her journey of self-discovery through vibrant, nutrient-rich meals. Her story unfolds like a recipe, each challenge met with a flavorful solution that not only nourished her body but also fed her soul.

Then there's Mike, who conquered the battle of the bulge by turning his kitchen into a sanctuary of wellness. His journey from fast food to flavorful, fat-burning recipes inspires, illustrating how small changes in culinary choices can yield remarkable results.

These stories are not just about weight loss; they are about reclaiming joy, celebrating health, and finding liberation through food. Each culinary triumph is a beacon, guiding readers towards their own successes. "Savoring Success" isn't merely a chapter; it's an invitation to savor the narratives of those who turned their kitchens into arenas of triumph, proving that the journey to a healthier, happier you is a saga worth savoring.

Chapter Five

Nutritional Alchemy For A Leaner You

In the alchemical realm of "Eat Your Food and Melt Body Fats," discover the enchanting secrets of "Nutritional Alchemy for a Leaner You." This chapter transcends conventional nutrition advice, weaving a tapestry of transformative culinary wisdom that reshapes your relationship with food.

Imagine your kitchen as a laboratory, each ingredient a mystical element in the process of crafting a leaner, healthier you. Unravel the mysteries of nutrient synergy as you indulge in the potion of protein-rich quinoa paired with vitamin-packed greens, a concoction that not only tantalizes your taste buds but also fuels your body's furnace.

Enter the alchemical dance of macronutrients, where the precise balance of healthy fats, lean proteins, and complex carbs becomes the elixir for sustained energy and satiety. Picture savoring the aromatic spell of metabolism-boosting spices, turning every meal into a potion that stirs the cauldron of fat-burning magic.

This isn't just a guide; it's an invitation to participate in the alchemy of your own well-being. Through these pages, witness the culinary transformation that transcends the mundane, where each meal becomes a step towards a leaner, more vibrant version of yourself. "Nutritional Alchemy for a Leaner You" is not just a chapter; it's a journey into the art of crafting meals that nourish, energize, and sculpt a healthier, alchemized you.

Chapter Six

Spice It Up: Herbs And Spices For Fat Loss

In the flavorful landscape of "Eat Your Food and Melt Body Fats," "Spice it Up: Herbs and Spices for Fat Loss" emerges as the tantalizing gateway to a culinary realm where every pinch, sprinkle, and dash transforms your plate into a palette of both pleasure and wellness.

Envision your kitchen as a spice bazaar, each jar holding the potential for a delicious metamorphosis. Dive into the seductive allure of cinnamon, not just a spice but a metabolism-boosting enchantress, transforming your morning oatmeal into a fragrant elixir that kick-starts your day.

Explore the fiery romance of cayenne pepper, a calorie-burning maestro that transforms mundane dishes into culinary masterpieces. Witness the herbaceous dance of rosemary, infusing roasted vegetables with not just flavor, but also antioxidants that nurture your body.

This isn't just a chapter; it's a symphony of aromas and tastes that elevate your culinary repertoire. Discover the secret language of herbs and spices, where every sprinkle tells a tale of both indulgence and fat-burning prowess. "Spice it Up" invites you to embrace the transformative power of spices, turning each meal into a celebration of health and flavor—a spice-filled journey towards a more vibrant, slimmer you.

Chapter Seven

Culinary Fitness: Crafting a Sustainable Meal Plan

"Culinary Fitness: Crafting a Sustainable Meal Plan" within the pages of "Eat Your Food and Melt Body Fats" is not a mere regimen; it's a symphony of flavors composing a sustainable lifestyle. Imagine your kitchen as a gym, and every meal a meticulously designed workout for your well-being.

Picture a meal plan as a personalized fitness routine, tailored to sculpt your body with the precision of a masterful trainer. Explore the vibrant variety of nutrient-rich foods, each ingredient selected not just for taste but as a powerhouse of sustenance. Engage in the harmonious balance of proteins, fats, and carbohydrates, creating a culinary equilibrium that fuels your journey to a leaner you.

As you delve into this chapter, witness the transformation of your plate into a canvas of nourishment. Embrace the versatility of plant-based proteins and the heartiness of whole grains, painting a portrait of energy and vitality. This isn't a restrictive diet; it's a celebration of mindful choices, transforming your kitchen into a realm of culinary fitness.

Crafting a sustainable meal plan becomes an art form, where each bite is a step towards a healthier, more robust version of yourself. "Culinary Fitness" isn't just a chapter title; it's an invitation to dance with flavors, creating a sustainable rhythm that resonates with the cadence of your well-being.

Chapter Eight

Indulge Wisely: Desserts For A Slimmer Waistline

In the delectable tapestry of "Eat Your Food and Melt Body Fats," "Indulge Wisely: Desserts for a Slimmer Waistline" is a sweet revelation, inviting you into a guilt-free confectionery haven where every dessert is not just a treat but a step towards a healthier you.

Imagine a dessert table adorned with dark chocolate-dipped strawberries, a decadent embrace of antioxidants and indulgence. Visualize savoring a creamy avocado chocolate mousse, where the richness is not just a delight to your taste buds but also a nod to smart, nutritious choices.

This chapter is a culinary alchemy, redefining the notion of desserts for weight management. Picture the dance of honey and Greek yogurt in a fruit parfait, sweetness that satisfies your cravings without compromising your waistline.

These desserts aren't a departure from your health goals; they're a delightful detour that keeps you on the path of wellness. "Indulge Wisely" transforms your sweet tooth into a compass guiding you towards desserts that not only please your palate but also contribute to your slimming journey. Dive into the art of crafting desserts that are both sinfully delicious and waistline-friendly, because in this confectionery narrative, every indulgence is a smart choice for a sweeter, slimmer you.

Chapter nine

Epilogue: Nourish, Melt And Thrive

In the crescendo of "Eat Your Food and Melt Body Fats," the epilogue, "Nourish, Melt, and Thrive," beckons readers into a transformative embrace of holistic well-being. Envision it as the final note in a symphony of culinary wisdom, resonating with the promise of a nourished, leaner, and thriving self.

This epilogue isn't just a farewell; it's an invitation to embark on a lifelong journey of mindful nourishment. Picture the satisfaction of savoring a well-balanced plate, where each ingredient not only delights your taste buds but also contributes to the ongoing masterpiece of your health.

Nourishment becomes the cornerstone, melting away the barriers to a healthier you. Envision the melting away of not just physical weight but also the burdens of dieting and self-doubt, leaving you free to revel in the joy of your culinary choices.

As the epilogue unfolds, the word "thrive" becomes a mantra. Visualize yourself not merely existing but flourishing, embodying vitality and wellness. It's an affirmation that your journey doesn't end with the last page; it evolves into a vibrant, ongoing symphony of health and happiness. "Nourish, Melt, and Thrive" is the resounding finale, echoing the promise that your culinary choices can be the catalyst for a life that's not just lived but exuberantly thrived.

Conclusion

In the final chapters of "Eat Your Food and Melt Body Fats," as readers embark on the journey toward a healthier, more vibrant life, they discover the transformative power of love – a love not only for oneself but also for the incredible journey of nourishing the body. The author delicately weaves a tapestry of words that goes beyond the mere act of consuming food; it becomes a dance with flavors, a symphony of nutrients that harmonize with the body's needs.

Through the pages, a unique romanticism emerges – a love affair with wholesome ingredients and the commitment to savoring each bite. The author guides readers towards a mindful appreciation of the culinary experience, turning ordinary meals into rituals of self-love. This love extends to the body, as the once-overlooked connection between food and emotion takes center stage, fostering a holistic approach to well-being.

The narrative crescendos as readers witness the constructive transformation of characters who not only shed physical weight but also liberate themselves from the burden of unhealthy habits. The author masterfully illustrates the parallel journey of self-discovery and self-love, intertwining romantic undertones with the empowering realization that true beauty emanates from within.

In the concluding pages, the readers find themselves immersed in a celebration of newfound vitality and confidence. The author leaves them with a tender reminder that the journey towards health is an ongoing love story – a commitment to nurturing the body, mind, and soul. As the last words linger, a sense of fulfillment envelops readers, inspiring them to savor not just the taste of their meals but the richness of life itself. The book concludes not just as a guide to melting body fats but as a testament to the profound connection between love, nourishment, and the art of living well.

9 798867 572631